Ki

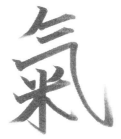

The Energy of Life

EDWARD ESKO

Words Using Ki

Ten Ki	Weather (Ki of heaven)
Ku Ki	Air (Ki of emptiness)
Gen Ki	Health (Original Ki)
Byo Ki	Sickness (Sick Ki)
Ki Chigai	Madness (Wrong Ki)
Yu Ki	Courage (Active Ki)
Ki ga Tsuku	Notice (Ki is focused)
Ki ga Kawaru	Change mind (Ki changed)
Ki ga Kiku	Clever (Ki works sharply)
Ki ga Noru	Want to do (Ki rides)
Ki ga Chisai	Coward (Ki is small)
Ki ga Shizumu	Depressed (Ki sinks down)
Ki ni Iru	Come to like (accepted in Ki)
Ki o Tsukau	Worry about (use Ki)
Jo Ki Suru	Excitement (Ki goes up high)
Ki o Tobasu	Frightened (Ki flies away)
Ki o Ushinau	Fall down unconsciously (Ki is lost)
Sho Ki	Sound judgment (Right Ki)
Ki Hin	Nobleness (Ki is good for three factors)
Uwa Ki	Womanizing (Ki is floating and wandering)

From Michio Kushi, *The Order of the Universe Magazine*, 1967

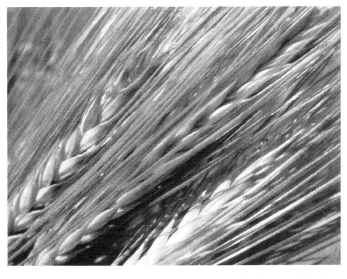

Cereal grains have the strongest Ki, or life energy, in the plant kingdom

KI
The Energy of Life

Contents

The Energy of Life   5
Chakras and Meridians   8
The Unity of Heaven and Earth   14
Ki in Daily Life   17
Reconnecting with Nature   24
Charts of the Meridians* 27
Meridians and Constellations   33

Resources   34
About the Author   35

KI The Energy of Life
From a lecture at the Kushi Institute
Calligraphy by Naomi Ichikawa
Edited by Noreen Dillman Purcell

Copyright © 2016 Edward Esko
ISBN-13: 978-1532727641
ISBN-10: 153272764X

*From *Basic Shiatsu*
Copyright © Michio Kushi and Edward Esko

Published by Amberwaves Press
P.O. Box 487
Becket, MA 01223
Amberwaves.org
Printed in the U.S.A.
First Edition

The Energy of Life

As Michio Kushi has pointed out in his lectures around the globe, life energy is called "Ki" in Japan, "Ch'i" in China, and "Prana" in India.

In Japan, the character for Ki (see below) is made up of two parts. The outer part depicts the entire universe coming into being and streaming out from infinity. It also depicts energy and the movement of the atmosphere. The inner part shows the image of a rice plant. You may notice that grains share a common characteristic. Tiny hair-like structures project from each grain. These are called "awns." The awns point toward the universe; they point upward to heaven. Like tiny antennae, they conduct energy or Ki from the cosmos. When we eat grain as our main food, we are receiving energy and information directly from the cosmos. That is why eating grain was thought to be essential for developing higher consciousness. Spiritual traditions around the world emphasized eating grain as the main food. That concept is symbolized in the character for Ki.

The inside lines show how the universe comes into being. As we can see, from infinity, or nothingness, represented by the blank white page, the initial manifestation is the appearance of two lines, one vertical and the other horizontal, or yin and yang. From the appearance of two opposite lines, another division occurs, so that two now become four. Four manifestations arise.

The four again divide, so that four become eight. Although not depicted in the character, eight then become sixteen; sixteen, thirty-two; thirty-two become sixty-four, etc., and so on to infinity. From one infinity arise infinite manifestations.

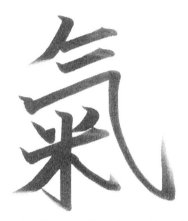

The character for "Ki." Calligraphy by Naomi Ichikawa

The process of division governs space and time. In the dimension of space, the directions north and south represent the initial division into two. They correspond to large yin and large yang. North and south then subdivide, producing west and east, or small yin and small yang. These are the four cardinal directions.

The four cardinal directions again divide, giving rise to the directions northeast, northwest, southeast, and southwest. In the dimension of time, the changing of the seasons follows the same pattern. We have two big opposite seasons that correspond to north and south. Winter corresponds to north and summer, to south; large yin and large yang.

Small yang corresponds to the direction east as does spring, and small yang to the direction west as does the autumn. In the twenty-four hour cycle of the day, north corresponds to nighttime, south to noon, east to morning, and west to sunset.

The character for Ki thus illustrates the universal pattern of creation. The timeless process of creation described in the character for Ki is also the foundation for the *Book of Changes* or *I Ching*. This several thousand-year-old book of cosmology, humanity, and society is one of the most revered in all of China. The concept of Ki is broad and vast. It adds a new dimension to our view of life. In western culture, this concept has largely been ignored, especially by modern medicine and science. It is only recently that the concept of life energy has emerged, spurred by contact with Asian culture. It is now appearing more and more in western countries. For hundreds of years, it was largely unknown.

Chakras and Meridians

Human life exists between two huge streams of energy. One is coming from the entire universe, pressing in on all sides toward the center of the earth. From our perspective this force is coming in. It appears to be pressing downward. Heaven's force originates in the infinite expansion and creates condensation, contraction, and density. Heaven's force spirals in and enters the top of the head. It animates the entire body and then exits from the lower body.

Meanwhile, because the earth is spinning, it gives off an opposite force. Earth's force originates from the core of the earth and spirals outward. It is outward, upward, and expanding. It produces diffusion, lightness, and dispersion. Heaven's force is pressing down; earth's force is expanding upward.

In the morning, earth's rising energy is predominant. So we get up and start our daily activity. The sun's energy hits the atmosphere and everything becomes active. At night, heaven's force takes over. Things quiet down and we lie down and go to sleep. Day and night, up and down, yin and yang. When we inhale, our body expands. When we stand up, we tend to inhale. When we sit down, we exhale. Heartbeat, digestive motion, and all of our bodily activities are animated by two basic energies: expansion and contraction, yin and yang.

On the earth, incoming energy enters at the poles. Energy entering at the North Pole collides with energy entering at the South Pole deep within the earth in the region known as the core. (Energy flows outward most strongly from the equator.) A highly charged energy center arises at the core, comprised of molten metals such as iron. This highly charged core is spinning and giving off electromagnetic energy that formed the various layers of the planet, such as mantle and crust. These layers radiate up toward the earth's surface and produce lines of energy. These highly charged lines create surface features. In North America, for example, one of these lines creates the Appalachian mountain range that runs from Maine to Georgia. Moving west, we have another highly charged range known as the Rocky Mountains. Even further west is the Sierra Nevada, and finally, one more range that hugs the Pacific Coast known as the Pacific Coastal Range. Mountain ranges correspond to the earth's meridians and are highly charged energy lines. They are produced by energy radiating up from the earth's highly charged core. This highly charged energy sometimes boils over producing a volcano.

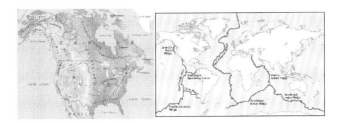

Earth's mountain ranges also exist deep below the ocean, for example, taking the form of the mid-Atlantic and mid-Pacific ranges. Energy lines also appear in the form of the borderlines between the earth's tectonic plates. These areas are also highly charged, so that when the earth's plates slip, a high-energy event known as an earthquake occurs.

Earth's energy doesn't stop at the surface, but radiates beyond the surface in the form of invisible energy lines that comprise the earth's magnetic field. This magnetic field radiates both toward and away from the sun.

This form is actually universal and found throughout nature. In vegetables and fruits we see a similar configuration. In a pumpkin, energy enters at its top through the stem. It forms the central area known as the core. The core is hollow. Highly charged seeds form in this hollow core. Each seed has the potential to sprout and grow into an entire organism. On its surface, we see ridges—energy lines radiating from the central core. A pumpkin has ridges, a cucumber has ridges, a squash has ridges, and a watermelon has ridges. These ridges are like the mountain ranges on the surface of the earth. Energy comes in, creates the core and radiates out toward the surface. The ridges are energy meridians. The core is known as a chakra. Our body has seven, the earth has one, and pumpkins have one. The human form is far more complex with seven chakras or energy centers.

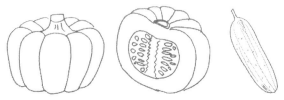

Illustration by Naomi Ichikawa

Not all vegetables have vertical meridians like those found on squash and pumpkins. Root vegetables like carrot, burdock, parsnip, and daikon have horizontal, not vertical meridians. Why is this so? Round vegetables channel energy from the earth through the stem at the top. This stem is connected to a vine that draws energy upward from the soil.

Tree fruits, like apples and pears, also have stems that connect to branches, trunks, and roots that channel earth's upward force. Thus their meridians take a more yin, vertical form. Because they are directly channeling earth's force, these fruits and vegetables assume a round shape like that of the earth, with a comparable core and meridian structure.

Root vegetables, on the other hand, channel heaven's yang downward force. As this force pushes downward from the sky to the earth, it encounters resistance from the dense and compact soil and from the upward, centrifugal energy generated by the earth's rotation. The energy of the root vegetable thus spirals around horizontally, like the threads on a drill. As it grows over time, the root burrows down into the soil.

Roots such as carrot, burdock, daikon, and dandelion are strongly charged with heaven's energy. As a whole, root vegetables are strongly polarized. They contain a dense and compact root portion, which branches downward, and a highly differentiated leafy portion that branches upward. Roots like daikon, turnip, and carrot normally have a single undivided root attached to a leafy top with many branches and leaves; they are a perfect example of balance between yang (root) and leaf (yin.)

In the human body, each chakra is responsible for a number of vital functions. The chakras are produced along the central core of energy. Similar to the earth's core and the pumpkin's core, our central core is where life energy is most powerful. We can live without a hand or an arm, but we cannot live without the central functions proximate to our core, including heart rhythm, absorption of nutrients, and brain function.

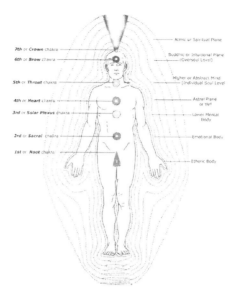

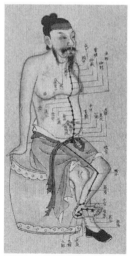

The seven chakras (above.) The kidney meridian (below)

In our body, we have the vertical energy channel that radiates upward and outward to the body's surface along invisible energy lines called meridians. There are twelve major meridians with approximately 365 highly charged points. The connection between our body and environment is clear. The meridians are like the ridges of the pumpkin or the mountain ranges of the earth. The human energy field does not end at the surface of the body, but radiates beyond the body in the form of invisible electromagnetic lines. That energy is especially charged above the head in what is known as the aura. The human aura corresponds to the earth's aura found above the poles which, at the North Pole, is known as the aurora borealis or "northern lights."

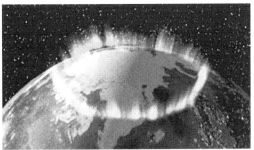

The northern lights or aurora borealis

The twelve meridians correspond to the twelve constellations, or groups of stars, circling the equator. In that sense they form a horizontal energy grid that creates balance with our vertical chakra channel. The twelve constellations are sending energy in horizontally toward the earth. These twelve streams pull energy up from the central line of chakras, forming the twelve meridians. When we study the chakras, meridians, points and their connections, we are actually studying the universe itself. The microcosm equals the macrocosm. As above, so below. We are the universe and the universe is us. The knowledge of Ki, or life energy, is the missing link in our understanding. It guides us in mapping the contours of this relationship.

The Unity of Heaven and Earth

If we have this energy form, how did we come to take material form? How did we materialize that energy body into physical form? For that, we need to understand how the universe takes form. It comes into being through what is known as fractal division. If we walk along a country road, we notice many types of vegetation, including different types of ferns. What is the pattern of the fern? The fern has one stem that divides into two, or yin and yang. Each division divides into two, and each new division further divides, in a continual pattern of one dividing into two, two dividing into four, four into eight, etc. That pattern continues again and again, extending upward and outward.

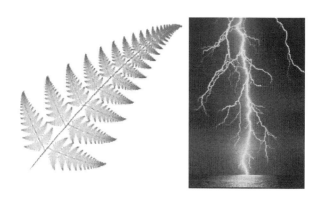

Fractals in nature

The same fractal division occurs in the body. Each meridian runs just below the surface of the body. The energy lines are like the ridges of the pumpkin running just below the skin line. Obeying the law of fractal division, branches come out from the main meridian channels. These branches continually divide, becoming smaller and smaller. At the end of each microscopic branch is a tiny spiral. Each of these spirals is a living cell.

The same thing occurs in our universe, in the macrocosmic world. There are giant streams of electromagnetic force, which extend across vast distances of outer space, in some cases more than a billion light years long. These energetic filaments are akin to the main meridian channels of the body. Like the meridians, they continuously subdivide. And, also like the meridians, at the end of each final subdivision are spirals of energy. From the point of view of the universe as a whole, these spirals are tiny, microscopic in scope. However, from our perspective, they are gigantic. Each spiral is actually a galaxy, like the Milky Way. Galaxies group together in clusters. These clusters are like groups of cells in our body, including specialized cells that form organs. Clusters of galaxies group together to form what are known as a "super cluster" of galaxies. Super clusters stretch across vast distances and are akin to our full body meridians or organ systems such as the digestive, respiratory, excretory, and nervous systems.

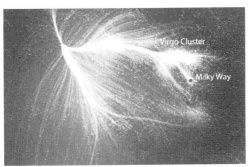

Computer model of galactic super-cluster

In his books and lectures Michio Kushi describes the human energy form, comprised of chakras, meridians, meridian branches, and cells, as the *Tree of Consciousness*. (The *Tree of Consciousness* may actually correspond to the *Tree of Life* mentioned in the Book of Genesis.) The *Tree of Consciousness* originates within the universe itself. Our physical body is created in the opposite way, from the material substance of the earth. The body is composed of minerals, proteins, fats, water, and air, arising from the world of elements found on earth. These elements continually replenish and enliven the body through food, drink, and breath. The nutrients in food are distributed to the entire body through the circulatory system, which is also formed through fractal division, as is life-giving oxygen. The large arteries that comprise the circulatory system continually branch into smaller and smaller vessels, at the end of which are microscopic capillaries that supply nutrients to the cells. The interface between the bloodstream, which is a fractal system, and the invisible energy form, also a fractal pattern, creates human life. We are the balancing point between heaven and earth.

Fractal patterns are the organizing principle of our body. We see that reflected clearly in the structure of the brain, the nervous system, the lungs and respiratory system, the heart and circulatory system and in the network of ducts in the liver, kidneys, pancreas, and other body structures. The human body is composed of multiple fractal systems, visible and invisible, physical and energetic, functioning as an integrated unit.

Ki in Daily Life

The secret to good health lies in maximizing the flow of energy through the body's visible and invisible channels. We can achieve this through diet and way of life. There are a number of practical methods for activating this life energy.

1. Diet

Whole grains contain strong life energy. With their outer husk intact, whole grains can survive for centuries and still sprout into living plants. This is why whole grains are essential to a healthy lifestyle. They contain life energy while milled grains or flour products, even when made from whole grains, do not. Whole grains like brown rice, barley, millet, and such are thus recommended for regular use. Their energetic qualities along with their nutrient density are the main reasons why whole grains are considered the principal food in the macrobiotic diet. (Refer to *The Book of Macrobiotics* for guidelines on an appropriate diet to maximize Ki flow.)

2. Cooking

Proper cooking is essential. Cooking adds energy to food and accelerates the release of energy and nutrients stored in foods. Cooking is a form of pre-digestion that helps break down plant fibers and release their stored energy and nutrients.

It is important to understand what cooking is. The body cannot easily assimilate tough plant fibers such as whole grains, beans, and many vegetables in their raw state. They are hard and tough. Cooking softens and makes them accessible. It is the first step in the breakdown of food into energy and nutrients. There is a great difference between human beings, who cook food, and wild animals that do not.

Have you seen the movie *Chimpanzee*? The chimps have their own culture and history. There are different tribes. The tribe featured in the film was in a good position. They lived around and controlled the nut grove. The chimps' main food was fruit, but fruit is lacking in protein. Nuts, which contain protein and fat, were an important supplement to their diet. The tribe that controlled the nut grove came under attack by a rival tribe who wanted to evict them. Incidentally, a diet of raw fruit and nuts is still deficient in protein. Because chimps are intelligent, they developed the ability to use tools to extract extra protein. So in the case of nuts, they learned how to crack the hard shells by striking them with a rock. The adults taught that skill to the younger chimps. To get more protein, they invented another method. They took a twig and stuck it down into an anthill. When they pulled it out, it was covered with ants, which they would eat for extra protein.

The chimps did not cook their food. They did not use fire. Their life is somewhat miserable and narrow compared to ours. When it rains, they must endure the cold and damp. They have no warmth and shelter. Plus their living space is small; their natural habitat is limited to a small section of the tropical forest, compared to the unlimited range of human settlement on the planet. There is a vast difference between humans and chimpanzees: grain eating versus no grain eating, the use of fire versus no fire.

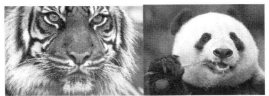

Yang (left) and yin (right.) The panda's teeth show that it may have eaten meat before it shifted to a bamboo diet

Incidentally, animals that eat primarily raw fruits and other raw plant foods are more yin than meat-eating carnivores. We can see that difference in the structure of their faces. Comparing a tiger to a panda, for example, we see that the tiger has eyes that slant upward, while the eyes of the panda slant downward. Upward slanting eyes are more yang, indicating a diet based more on animal food and an aggressive nature. Eyes that slant downward show a plant-based diet and a more passive disposition. The panda's main food is bamboo, a yin rapidly growing plant. This is why pandas, especially those in captivity, are lackadaisical about performing yang functions including mating and reproduction. The human face, which developed from eating grain, is between these extremes.

3. Method of Cooking

The method we use to cook our foods has a profound effect on our energy. Cooking over a wood or gas flame activates life energy, while electric cooking or microwaving diminishes or even destroys this energy. A gas flame is an extension of our fingers. It allows for the flexible adjustment of the heat we use in each step of the cooking process. It responds immediately to touch. Electric cooking does not allow such flexibility and immediacy of response.

4. Chewing

Another important practice for strengthening life energy is to chew our food well.

We can understand our digestion in terms of physical, biochemical reactions or in terms of energy, or in terms of both physical and energetic reactions. The enzymes in the mouth are essential in the digestion of grains. Mixing food with these enzymes when we chew sets in motion the active and efficient processes of digestion that follow. It is essential to the proper breakdown and absorption of our foods.

Not only does saliva contain enzymes essential for digestion, it is also highly charged with Ki or life energy. As we saw earlier, heaven's force enters the body at the top of the head. It flows downward toward the mouth, initially forming the uvula. Meanwhile, also in the mouth, earth's upward energy enters and forms the tongue. Branching downward and to the left and right of the uvula are two highly energized spirals. These spirals form the salivary glands. The thick liquid secreted there is highly energized. Thus, saliva has energizing and healing properties and initiates the breakdown and release of the energy in our foods.

5. Upright Posture

When we eat, we normally maintain an upright, vertical posture, usually sitting. The digestion of food utilizes heaven's downward energy that charges the body when we are standing or sitting upright. Food moves downward through the digestive tract. This force becomes much weaker when we lie down and sleep. Our digestion becomes sluggish and inefficient when we assume a horizontal position. Additional energy is required to break down and absorb the nutrients in food. Therefore it is important not to eat before going to bed, ideally for about 2 ½ to 3 hours.

If you go out late at night for pizza, you will feel sluggish the next morning. It is hard to get out of bed. Digestion is improper. At night we lie down and expose our body to the energy of the universe in the night sky.

Nighttime is the time of recharging, like recharging your cellphone. Normally we receive energy from the universe. It is the time for taking in Ki and using it for healing and regeneration. Healing occurs at night. If you have to use energy for digestion, you are taking it away from healing and regeneration, making it harder to recover from illness.

6. Daily Walking

Walking activates your Ki, charging your body with heaven and earth's forces. Walking and other forms of activity strengthen all functions such as breathing, circulation, appetite, digestion, mental clarity and the ability to discharge. It is ideal to walk in natural surroundings, especially surrounded by trees and other vegetation, which provide oxygen. Walking along a freeway is not as beneficial. A daily ½ hour walk is especially recommended.

7. Walking Barefoot

Many years ago, Michio Kushi added the suggestion to walk barefoot whenever safe and appropriate, for example on clean, unpolluted, and tick-free grass, soil, or beach. The reason is that contact with the earth stimulates the flow of beneficial energy we receive from the planet.

According to current theory, the earth is a huge electrically charged body, something like a giant battery. Nonstop lightning striking the surface (an estimated 5,000 strikes per minute), the movements of its interior, and the rotation of the planet itself are constantly charging it. The earth has an excess of free electrons and a net negative charge.

On the other hand, energy coming from the sun and other celestial bodies is positively charged. This theory is in accord with the macrobiotic classification of earth's force as yin (negative) and heaven's force as yang (positive.)

In general, for optimal health it is important to maintain an active flow of more yin energy, including an ample supply of free electrons from the surface of the earth. One way to accomplish this is to base the diet primarily on plant foods, which are strongly charged with earth's rising energy, while using animal food, which is a concentrated form of yang, heaven's energy, as an occasional supplementary food.

Another way to maintain health is to have regular contact with the earth by walking barefoot. Free electrons (yin) are taken up through the feet and have the effect of neutralizing immune stimulating, inflammation-producing, and cell-damaging free radicals, which are molecules that lack electrons and have a net positive charge. When the body is lacking in free electrons, it picks them up from the earth's surface, thus easing inflammation and free radical damage. Free electrons also have the effect of reducing harm caused by an excess of cortisol, a stress-inducing hormone. Cortisol, which is yang, is more abundant during the day (yang) and less so at night (yin.) We can summarize these effects as follows:

Imbalance	Neutralizing Factor
Heaven's force (yang)	Earth's force (yin)
Animal food	Plant food
Lack of contact with the earth	Contact with the earth
Free radicals (positive)	Free electrons (negative)
Cell damage	Cell regeneration

Earth's energy, or Ki, including the free electrons described above, flows into the body especially through the point at the bottom of the foot known as Kidney 1. This point is the beginning of the kidney meridian that flows up the inside of the leg and up the front of the body.

The kidney meridian connects with the bladder meridian, which flows in the opposite direction, from the head down the back and the back of the leg to the fifth toe (refer to the meridian charts in the following section.) The bladder meridian has sets of points, known as Yu points that connect to all the major organs. Energizing the kidney and bladder meridians stimulates all the major organs and functions and is one benefit of walking barefoot.

8. Activating the Skin

Dry brushing or scrubbing the body with a hot wet towel is beneficial to activate life energy. The modern diet high in animal protein and fat makes the skin become hard and dry, almost like the skin of a steer. What are the effects on our health? The skin is the largest organ of discharge. If excess can't go out, but instead is discharged internally, sickness arises. It is important to keep the skin soft and supple, so that discharge can take place smoothly. Activating the skin also stimulates circulation and the flow of energy along the meridians.

Related to that is the practice of removing callus from the feet and toes. Callus represents the discharge of protein and fat, especially from animal food. Callus typically occurs on the outside of the large toe, in the area corresponding to the liver and pancreas. It blocks the flow of energy through these meridians. Callus on the heel corresponds to blockage or stagnation in the sexual organs. It is important to remove callus either through rubbing with a stone or visiting the nail salon. Soaking both feet in hot water before bed not only helps you to sleep more soundly but also helps soften hard callus and is highly recommended.

Reconnecting with Nature

Artificial lights raise night sky luminance, creating the most visible effect of light pollution—artificial sky-glow. Despite the increasing interest among scientists in fields such as ecology, astronomy, health care, and land-use planning, light pollution lacks a current quantification of its magnitude on a global scale. To overcome this, we present the world atlas of artificial sky luminance, computed with our light pollution propagation software using new high-resolution satellite data and new precision sky brightness measurements. This atlas shows that more than 80% of the world and more than 99% of the U.S. and European populations live under light-polluted skies. The Milky Way is hidden from more than one-third of humanity, including 60% of Europeans and nearly 80% of North Americans. Moreover, 23% of the world' s land surfaces between 75°N and 60°S, 88% of Europe, and almost half of the United States experience light polluted nights. —The New World Atlas of Artificial Night Sky Brightness, Science Advances, June 2016

Modern medicine, with all of its incredible analytical devices, could not discover the body's energy system. It remained elusive. How did ancient people detect and map the body's energy system?

Ancient people must have been very intuitive, sensitive, and in tune with nature and the universe. Ancient astronomy was highly developed, for example, in Babylonia and among the Egyptians and Chinese. The same is true with their architecture, including the pyramids in Egypt, Mexico, and China.

Ancient people ate a natural diet that was locally and seasonally based. They ate whole grains that helped orient their consciousness toward the universe itself. As we saw, whole grains have antennae that point toward the cosmos. As a result they were sensitive to the cosmos and could feel and detect this natural energy or Ki. They also were living much closer to nature. How does that compare with people today? The modern diet is highly processed and unnatural. It dulls, rather than enhances, sensitivity to nature.

Modern cities also cut people off from the natural environment. They are certainly exciting and fun, but are not especially in tune with nature. How about the difference between day and night? As the study quoted above demonstrates, light pollution is blocking natural energy, especially starlight at night. Day and night are less vivid in the city as compared to the countryside, where day and night are more clearly differentiated. How about the seasons? Winter, spring, summer, and fall are not so different in the city. Air conditioning and central heating remove us from natural conditions, as does the proliferation of electronic devices. These devices block natural energy.

Not long ago, I was taking the Long Island ferry across Long Island Sound. It was a beautiful clear sunny day. The surroundings were perfect. A young couple with two teenaged kids boarded the ferry. They were tourists. Like me, the parents were enjoying the beautiful natural surroundings. The two kids, a boy and girl, didn't look up once. They were busy texting. They didn't even see the beauty around them. They could have cared less. Clearly, we are losing touch with our natural environment and the natural flow of energy both within and without.

The simple suggestions presented in this booklet, eating a natural diet centered on whole grains and other plant foods, keeping active, and reconnecting with nature are all designed to help strengthen your health and well being while enhancing the flow of life energy throughout your body and mind.

Charts of the Meridians

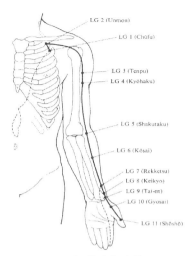

Lung (LG) Meridian

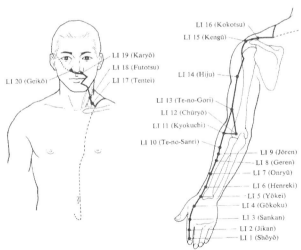

Large Intestine (LI) Meridian

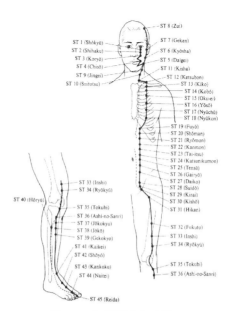

Stomach (ST) Meridian

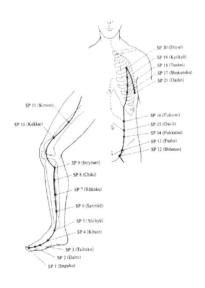

Spleen (SP) Meridian

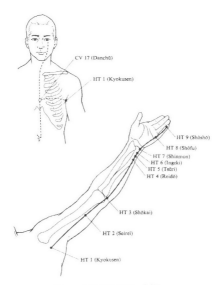

Heart (HT) Meridian

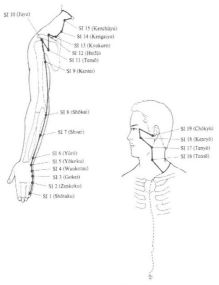

Small Intestine (SI) Meridian

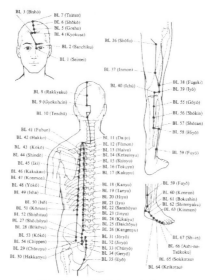

Bladder (BL) Meridian

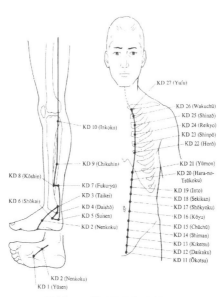

Kidney (KD) Meridian

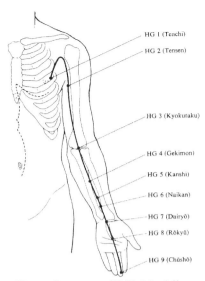

Heart Governor (HG) Meridian

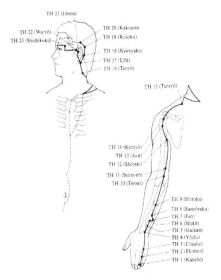

Triple Heater (TH) Meridian

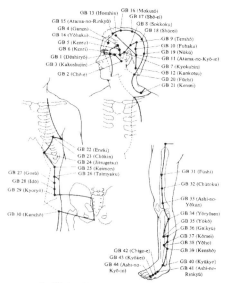

Gallbladder (GB) Meridian

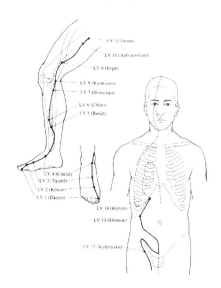

Liver (LV) Meridian

Meridians and Constellations

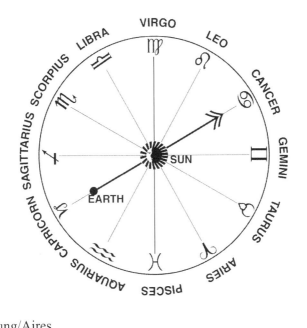

Lung/Aires
Large Intestine/Taurus
Stomach/Gemini
Spleen/Cancer
Heart/Leo
Small Intestine/Virgo
Bladder/Libra
Kidney/Scorpio
Heart Governor/Sagittarius
Triple Heater/Capricorn
Gallbladder/Aquarius
Liver/Pisces

Resources

Kushi Institute, 198 Leland Road, Becket MA 01223, 413-623-5741, www.kushiinstitute.org. World Center for Macrobiotic Learning. Programs include the Way to Health Residential Seminar, Macrobiotic Leadership Training, Specialty Workshops, and the annual Kushi Summer Conference. Programs presented by the world's leading macrobiotic teachers and educators. The Kushi Institute sponsors a natural products store with mail order books, CDs, and videos by the author plus a range of high-quality macrobiotic foods. Visit KushiStore.com.

Planetary Health/Amberwaves, PO Box 487, Becket MA 01223, 413-623-0012, www.amberwaves.org. A grassroots network devoted to preserving amber waves of grain and keeping America and the planet beautiful. Amberwaves is publisher of numerous books and a quarterly newsletter with articles by Edward Esko and Alex Jack.

***Macrobiotics Today*/George Ohsawa Macrobiotic Foundation (GOMF)**, 1277 Marian Ave., Chico CA 95928, 800-232-2372, www.OhsawaMacrobiotics.com. GOMF is a macrobiotic publisher and educational center on the West Coast. *Macrobiotics Today* quarterly features articles by Edward Esko and other macrobiotic authors.

About the Author

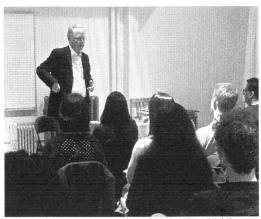

Photo of the author in New York City by Naomi Ichikawa

Edward Esko is one of the world's most active contemporary macrobiotic teachers. Over the past four decades, he has lectured and counseled in Europe, Asia, Latin America, and throughout North America, including at the United Nations, and has written and edited numerous books and articles. Building on the teachings of George Ohsawa, Michio Kushi, and other macrobiotic pioneers, he has applied yin and yang—the universal principles of change and harmony—to helping solve issues of personal and planetary health. He has served as Vice President of the East West Foundation. He currently serves as Associate Director and Senior Faculty member at the Kushi Institute. His latest books include *Yin Yang Primer, Contemporary Macrobiotics, Rice Field Essays,* and *Dandelion Essays*, as well as *Cool Fusion* and *Corking the Nuclear Genie,* coauthored with Alex Jack. Books are available from amazon and KushiStore.com. Contact: edwardesko@gmail.com.

Printed in Great Britain
by Amazon